YOUR KNOWLEDGE HAS VALUE

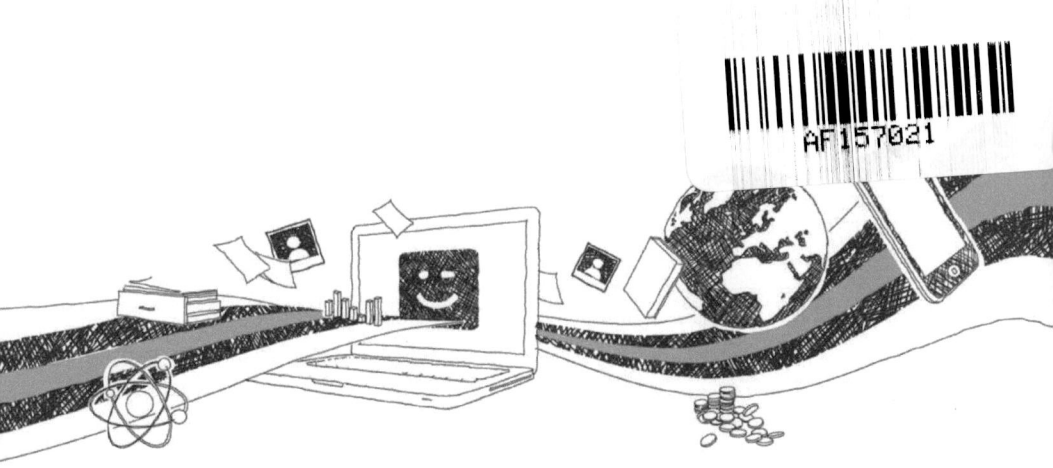

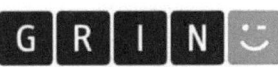

Bibliographic information published by the German National Library:

The German National Library lists this publication in the National Bibliography; detailed bibliographic data are available on the Internet at http://dnb.dnb.de .

Imprint:

Copyright © 2019 GRIN Verlag
Print and binding: Books on Demand GmbH, Norderstedt Germany
ISBN: 9783668989290

This book at GRIN:

https://www.grin.com/document/486923

Robert Vollmann

Magnetic resonance imaging for initial diagnosis of sporadic Creutzfeldt Jakob disease

Case series and review

GRIN Verlag

GRIN - Your knowledge has value

Since its foundation in 1998, GRIN has specialized in publishing academic texts by students, college teachers and other academics as e-book and printed book. The website www.grin.com is an ideal platform for presenting term papers, final papers, scientific essays, dissertations and specialist books.

Visit us on the internet:

http://www.grin.com/

http://www.facebook.com/grincom

http://www.twitter.com/grin_com

Table of contents

Magnetic resonance imaging for initial diagnosis of sporadic Creutzfeldt Jakob disease

Abstract:

Sporadic Creutzfeldt–Jakob disease (sCJD) is a fatal neurodegenerative disorder caused by expression of abnormal human prion proteins in the brain. sCJD causes rapidly progressive dementia (RPD). For a definitive diagnosis, brain biopsy or autopsy is required (definite CJD). Premortally diagnosed patients are called probable CJD according to the diagnostic criteria of Zerr et al.

The aim of this case series is to show the reliability of magnetic resonance imaging (MRI) in the initial diagnosis of this disease compared to other diagnostic modalities. Furthermore we give a review of literature to confirm our observations.

Our case series consisted of six patients; four were diagnosed with definite sCJD and two with probable sCJD.

Diffusion weighted imaging (DWI), EEG and cerebrospinal fluid (CSF) was examined in all patients.

All patients showed diffusion restriction in the basal ganglia and/or cortex in DWI and CSF analysis was positive for 14-3-3 protein in five patients. EEG showed typical changes in three cases. The clinical examination revealed heterogenic results. One patient had typical MRI changes even present before the onset of symptoms.

Our case series and a literature review showed that DWI with ADC map are a highly sensitive and specific tools for the initial diagnosis of sCJD especially when clinical features appear atypical for the disease.

Introduction:

CJD is a very rare entity with an incidence of one in two millions. It is an infectious disease caused by abnormal proteins, which are called prions (1).

The so called prion hypothesis describes a transformation from the normal cellular prion protein into the pathologic form called scrapie, which tends to accumulate and induces neuronal cell death and spongiform changes of the brain (1).

Four different forms of CJD are known: the sporadic type (sCJD), the genetic type, the iatrogenic type and the variant type. Prion diseases have a fatal prognosis and no treatment exists (2).

We focused here on the most common form of prion disease: sCJD. Most patients with sCJD are about 60 – 70 years old. They typically present with RPD and focal neurologic signs including ataxia, pyramidal and extrapyramidal disorders or visual disturbances (2). The mean duration of the disease is 6 months with a range from several weeks up to two years (3).

Electroencephalogram (EEG) and the analysis of cerebrospinal fluid (CSF) may be helpful in the diagnosis. EEG shows periodic sharp wave complexes (PSWC) in about two thirds of sCJD patients (4).

The 14-3-3 protein is a neuronal protein which is released into the CSF as a result of extensive destruction of the brain tissue and therefore, this protein is also an important parameter for the detection of sCJD (5).

MRI has been proven to be a very powerful tool in the premortal diagnosis of CJD (6).

However the main problem is that a definite diagnosis can only be made by the autopsy report. According to the updated diagnostic criteria by Zerr et al (7), premortal probable sCJD is determined when two of the following four clinical features are met: 1. dementia, 2. visual or cerebellar signs, 3. pyramidal or extrapyramidal signs, 4. acinetic mutism. Additionally at least one of the following laboratory tests must be positive: 1. typical EEG (periodic sharp wave complexes), 2. detection of 14-3-3 protein in CSF in patients that suffer from sCJD for less than two years; and 3. MRI signal abnormalities in DWI or fluid attenuated inversion recovery (FLAIR)

The aim of this case series is to show the reliability of MRI in the initial diagnosis of CJD. The exact and early diagnosis is essential to exclude other treatable diseases.

Materials and Methods:

Patient's characteristics:

The institutional review board approved this HIPPA compliant retrospective study; patient informed consent was waived.

A database search including the term Creutzfeldt Jakob disease revealed the names of twelve patients during the last ten years. We had to exclude five patients due to the lack of MRI data. Another patient was excluded because of genetic CJD. All patients had a negative history of familial diseases or exposure to known prion-contaminated, neurosurgical instruments, tissue grafts, and pituitary extracted hormones.

This case series consists of six patients, four females and two male. Four patients were diagnosed with definite sCJD and two with probable sCJD according to the updated diagnostic criteria.

DWI was available in all of them. Furthermore all patients received EEG and CSF examination for 14-3-3 protein.

Imaging Characteristics:

We performed MRI examinations with a 1.5 Tesla system (Siemens Magnetom Espree). The imaging protocol included a DW single-shot spin echo echoplanar sequence acquired in the anterior commissure-posterior commissure (diffusion gradient b values of 0 and 1000 s/mm^2, repetition time [TR] 5000 ms, echo time [TE] 114 ms, slice thickness 6 mm with no gap, matrix of 192x100 pixels, and field of view of 230 mm); fluid-attenuated inversion recovery (FLAIR; TR/TE 9770/99 ms, inversion time 2200 ms); and T2-weighted turbo spin echo sequences (TR/TE 4500/85 ms). For diffusion weighted MRI, the diffusion gradients were successively and separately applied in 3 orthogonal directions for a total acquisition time of 97 seconds. Trace images were then generated and ADC maps were calculated with dedicated software tool (Syngo; Siemens).

Data Acquisition: MRI scans were interpreted by an experienced neuroradiologist. We reviewed the medical history for clinical examination, CSF analysis and EEG. Furthermore we compared our findings with a review of literature.

Case 1

A 70-year-old female patient   was transferred to hospital because of vertigo. The first symptoms appeared three weeks ago. The initial clinical examination revealed ataxia. The patient was initially orientated and no cognitive impairment was detectable. MRI revealed restricted diffusion in the cortex of the occipital, frontal and temporal lobe on the left side and the left sided caudate nucleus (Fig. 1). No changes have been detected on FLAIR and T2w sequences. EEG showed PSWC on the left hemisphere of the brain.

Within the next weeks, a rapid deterioration and cerebellar symptoms could be detected. The patient developed a rapidly progressive dementia.

CSF analysis was positive for 14-3-3 protein. According to these results the patient was diagnosed with probable sCJD. The patient died 37 days after the initial diagnosis. The autopsy of the brain confirmed the diagnosis of sCJD.

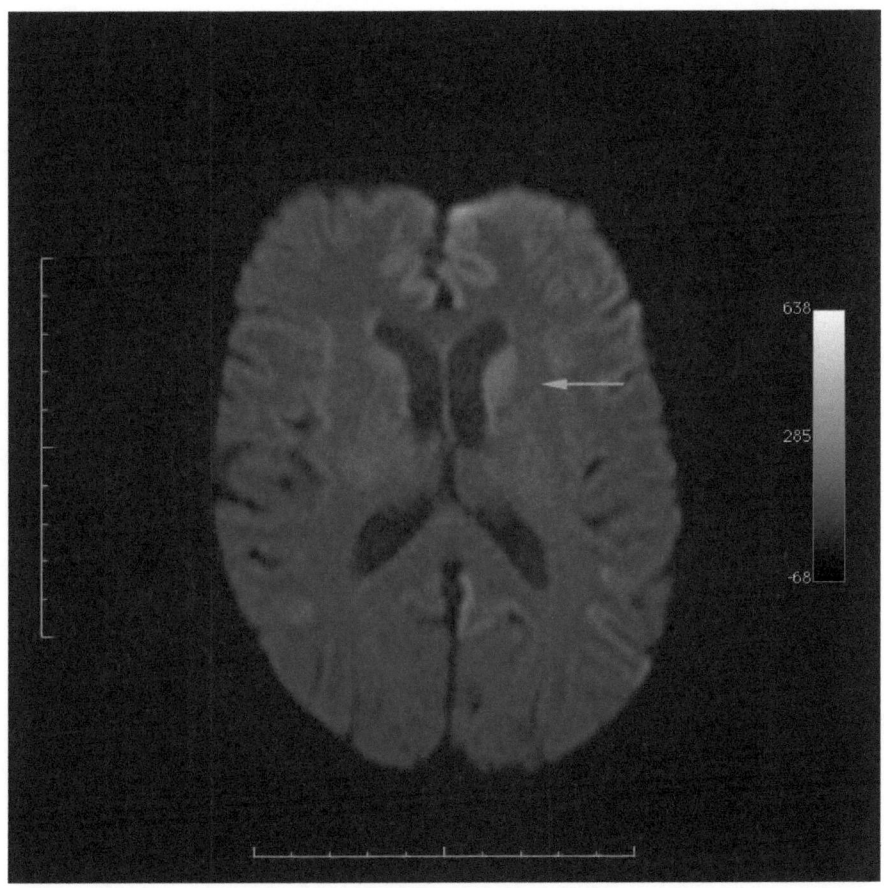

Fig. 1: DWI reveals high signal in the left caudate nucleus (arrow) and slightly

in the cortical regions of the frontal and temporal lobe.

Case 2

We report a 52-year-old female patient who was admitted to hospital because of tremor and changed mental status. The onset of symptoms was three months ago. Furthermore the patient suffered from dysphagia and ataxia.

MRI revealed symmetric restriction of diffusion in the caudate nucleus, putamen, thalami and cortical in the frontal and temporal lobes (Fig. 2 and Fig. 3). FLAIR sequence showed high signal in putamen and caudate nucleus (Fig. 4). CSF analysis was positive for 14-3-3 protein but EEG examination did not show any clear lesions. However, the patient fulfilled the criteria for probable sCJD. She deteriorated within a few weeks and could not swallow anymore. So a percutaneous endoscopic gastrostomy (PEG) was performed. The patient did not show up for follow up examination. Autopsy was not available in this case.

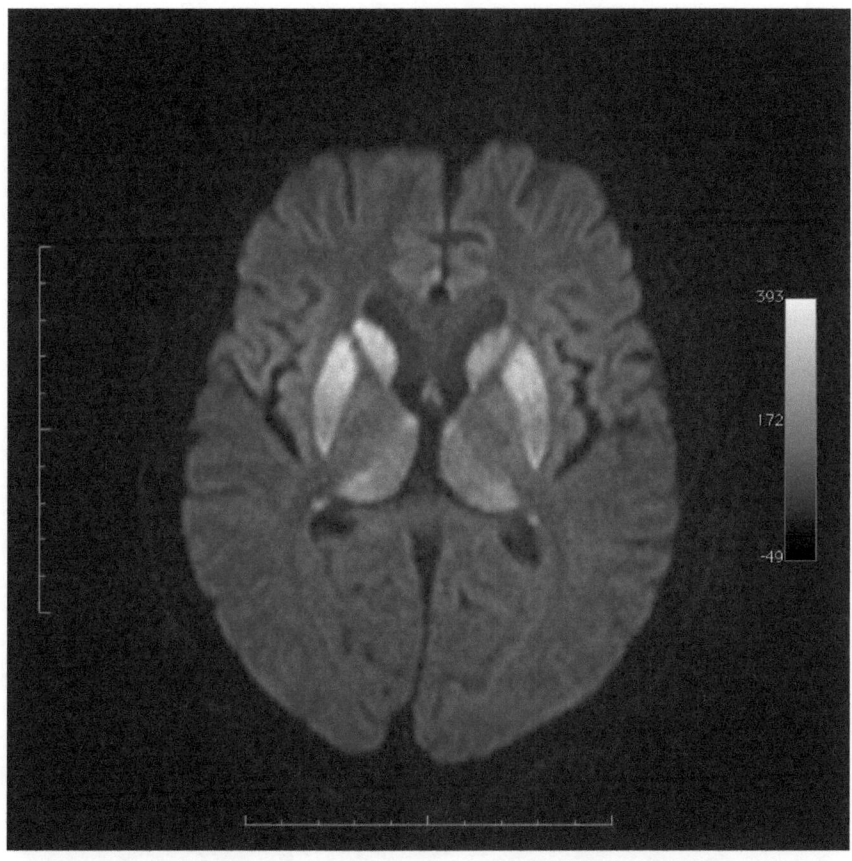

Fig. 2: DWI with symmetric hyperintense signal alteration in the putamen,

caudate nucleus and thalami.

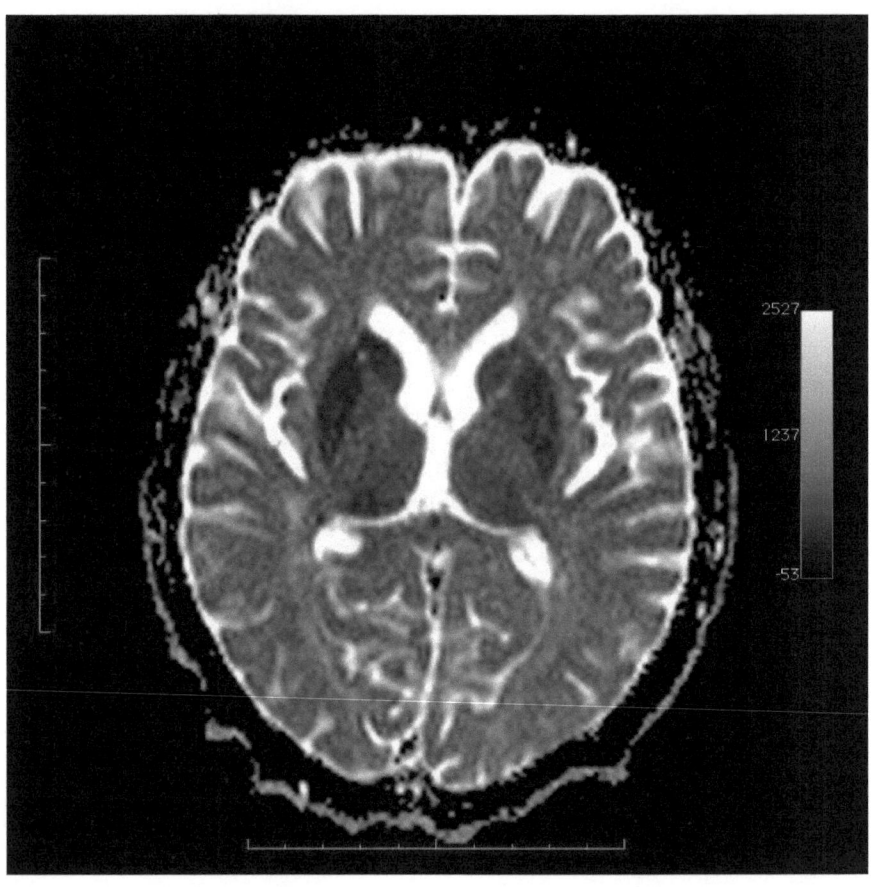

Fig. 3: ADC map same patient as Fig. 2. Low signal in the puatmen, caudate
nucleus and also in the thalami, which is an almost pathognomonic pattern for
sCJD.

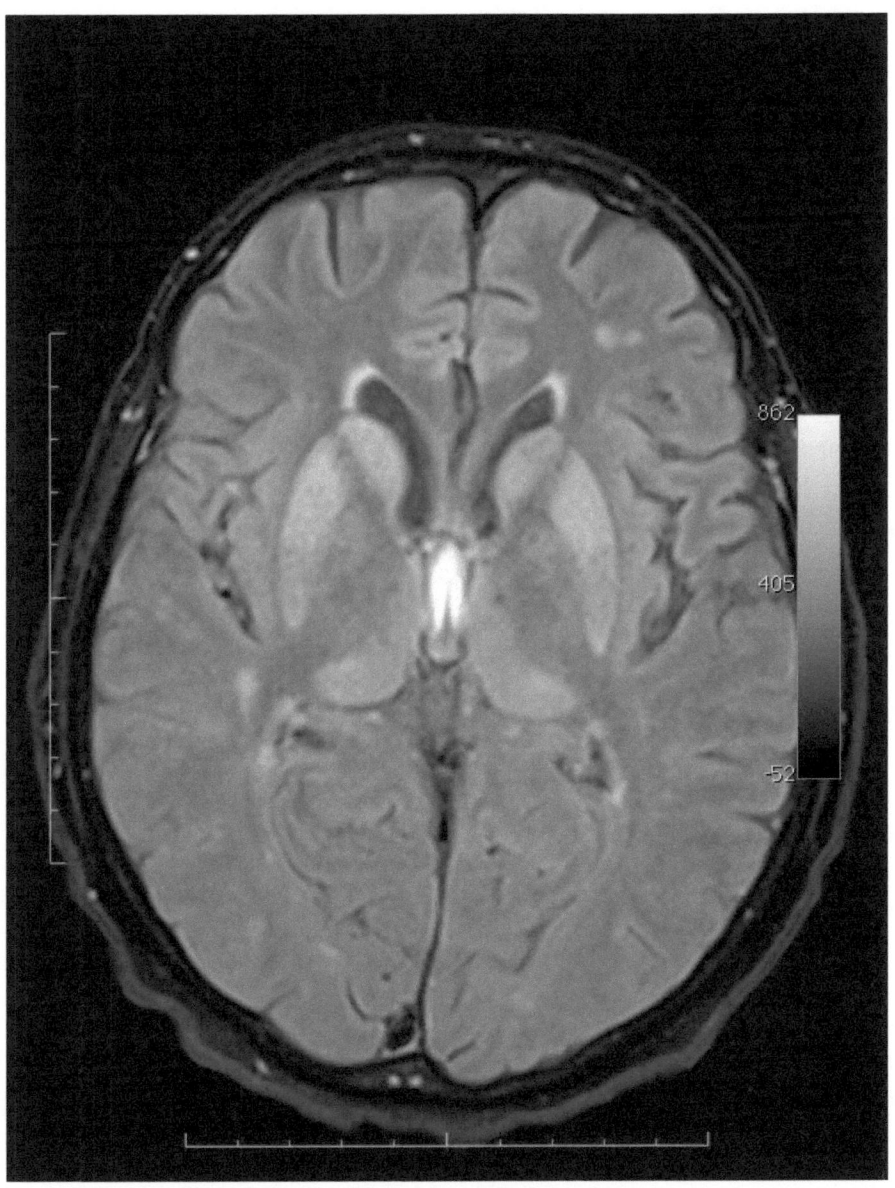

Fig. 4: Same patient as Fig. 2 and 3. FLAIR sequence also demonstrates the same changes seen on DWI.

Case 3

This 62-year-old male patient was transferred to hospital because of RPD and
hemianopsia. The symptoms started four weeks ago and worsened. MRI
revealed restricted diffusion in the cortex in the parietal lobe on the right and the
left sided temporal lobe (Fig. 5). FLAIR and T2w sequences did not
demonstrate abnormal signal in the cortex. EEG showed PSWC. CSF analysis
was also positive for the 14-3-3 protein. Taken together, this patient fulfilled the
diagnostic criteria for probable sCJD.

60 days after the initial diagnosis the patient died and autopsy confirmed
postmortally definitive sCJD.

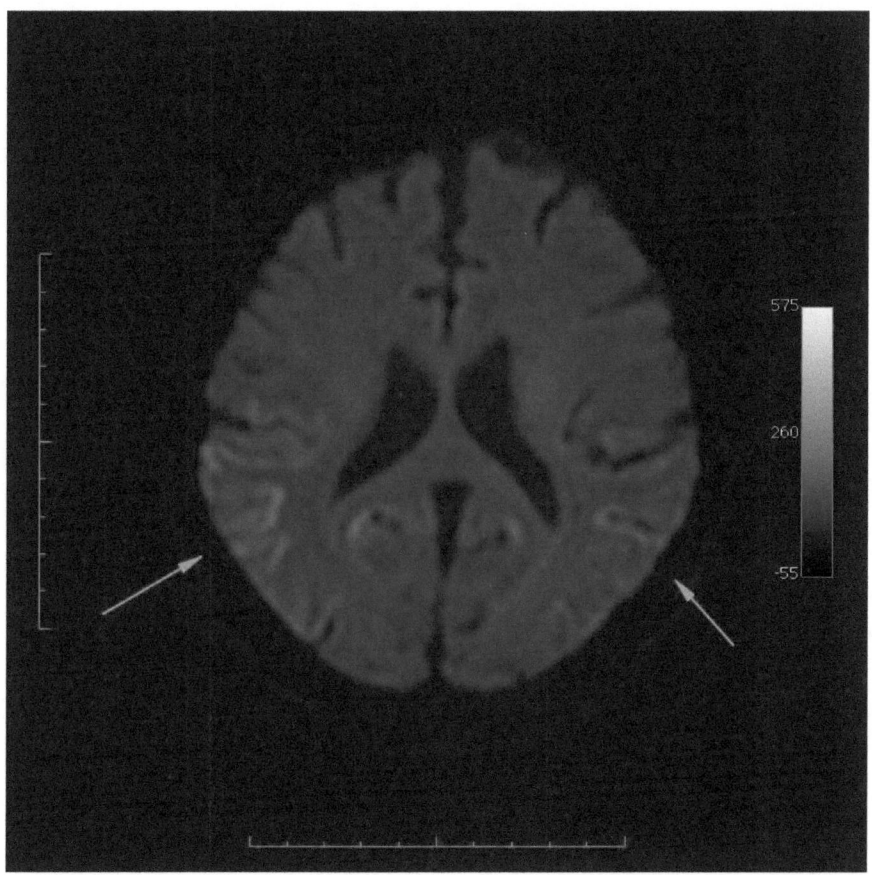

Fig. 5: Cortical hyperintense signal alteration in the cortical regions (arrow).
Note the typical sparing of the visual cortex.

Case 4

61-year-old female patient was admitted to the hospital because of tremor,
which had started at least five years ago. Despite medical treatment the tremor

remained. There was no cognitive impairment at the time of admission. Besides the tremor the clinical examination revealed no abnormalities.

The patients claimed that she just wanted to eat sweet food and nothing else, which was unusual for her according to the family.

The MRI revealed restricted diffusion in the thalamus and putamen and caudate nucleus (Fig. 6 and Fig. 7). High signals in these regions have also been detected by FLAIR (Fig. 8). EEG remained normal and 14-3-3 protein was negative. The criteria for sCJD in this patient were not fulfilled and because of the clinical examination a prion disease was not a likely diagnosis. A follow up MRI examination 17 days later revealed no changes compared to the initial findings.

The patient deteriorated within the next few weeks. She was not able to walk and talk anymore. 50 days after admission to hospital the patient died. The patient's autopsy confirmed sCJD.

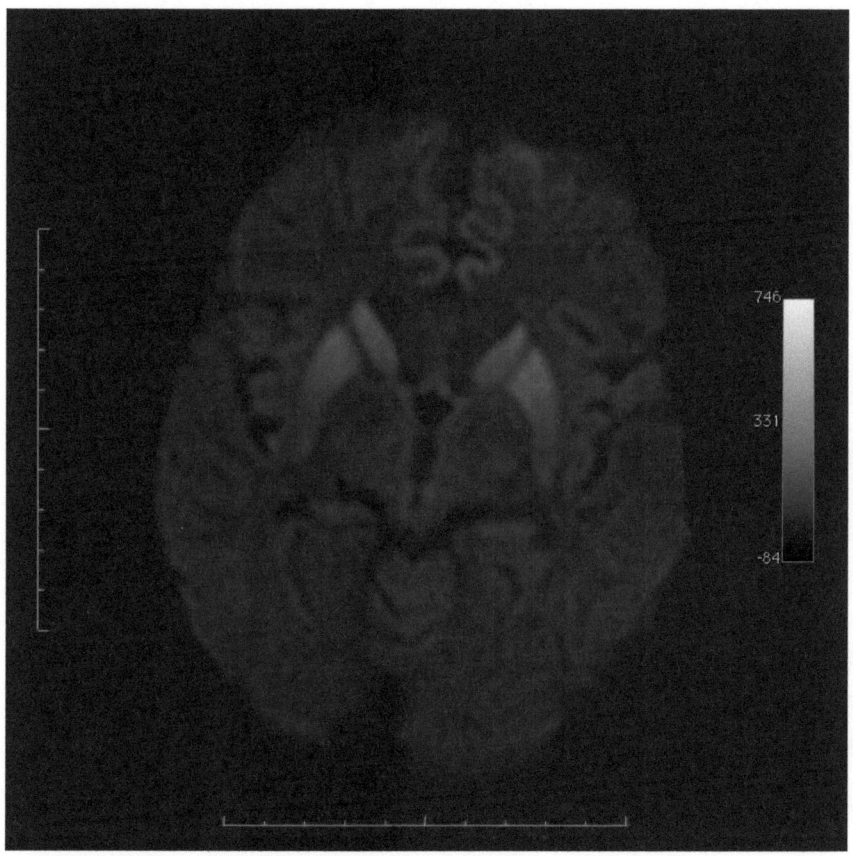

Fig. 6: DWI reveals typical signal changes in the caudate nucleus and putamen on both sides, which typiacally appear in sCJD.

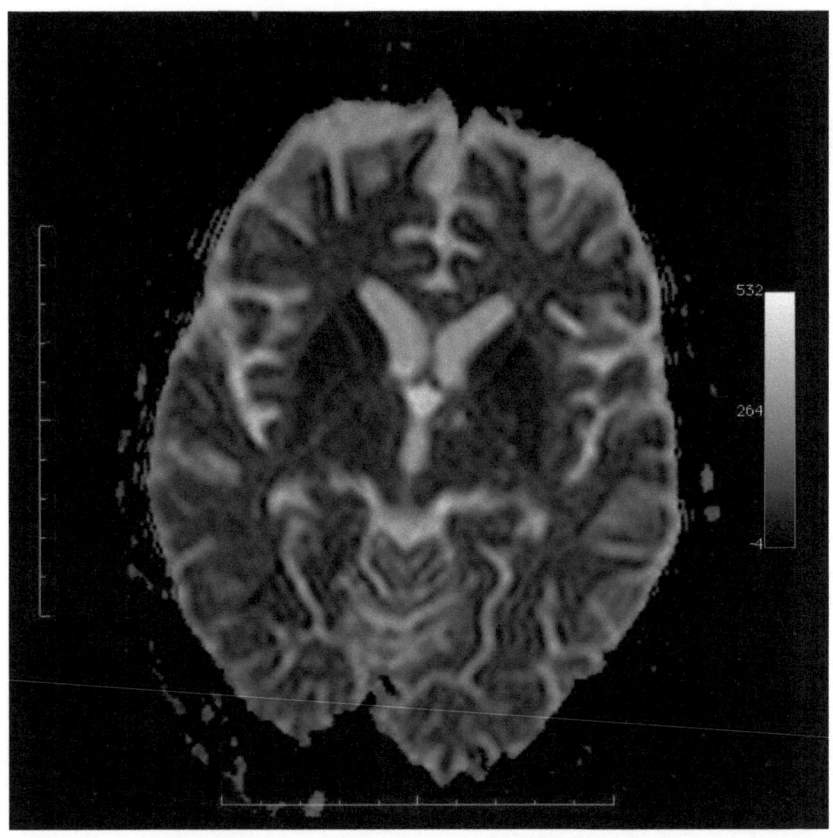

Fig. 7: ADC map from the same patient seen in Fig. 6. Symmetric restricted

diffusion in the caudate nucleus and putamen with low values at ADC map.

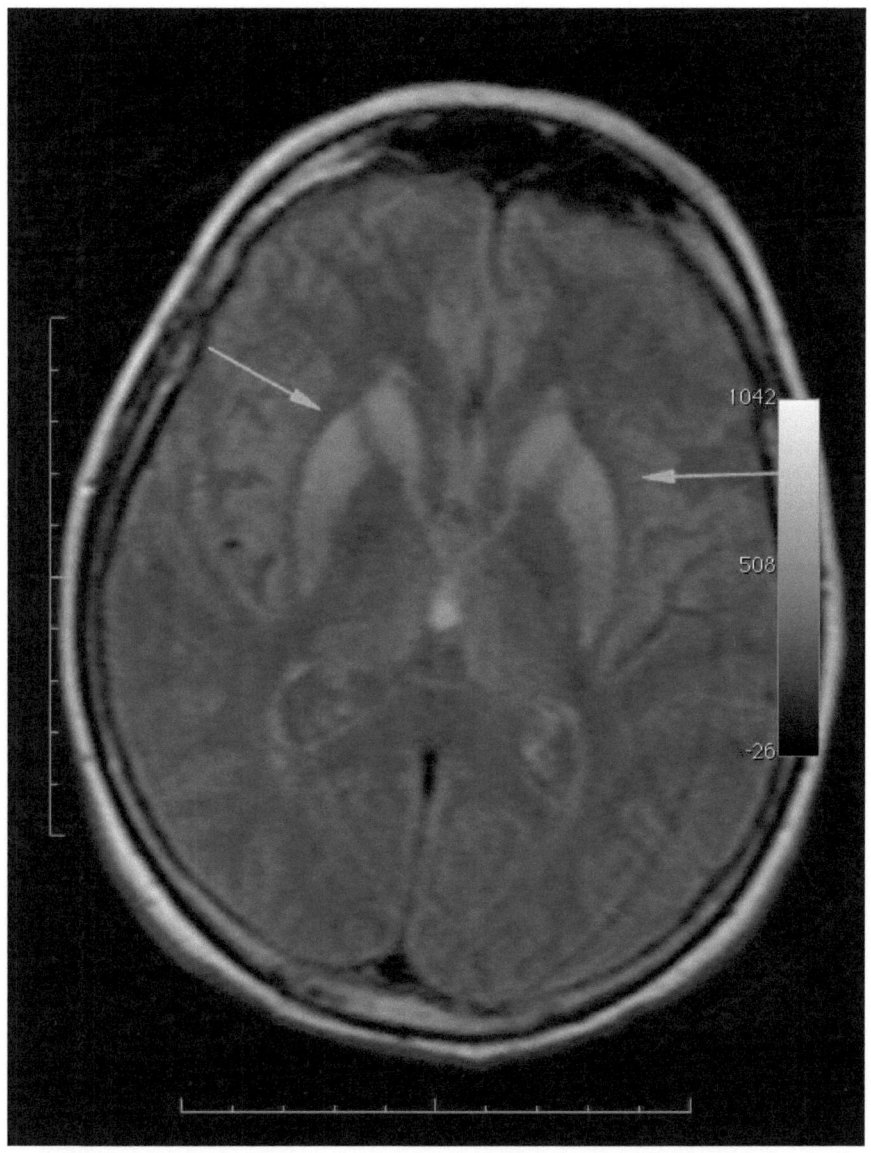

Fig. 8: Same patient as Fig 6 and 7. FLAIR sequence also reveals signal
alterations on the same locations seen on DWI and ADC map.

Case 5

This 75-year-old male patient was transferred to hospital due to rapidly progressive dementia and weakness of his left hand. Because of altered mental status a conversation with the patient was not possible.

The patient's son claimed that his father did not show any abnormalities two weeks earlier.

The MRI revealed diffusion restriction in the putamen, caudate nucleus and the right-sided cortex of the temporal lobe (Fig. 9). FLAIR also detected hyperintense lesions in the putamen and caudate nucleus. EEG revealed typical PSWC. CSF analysis was positive for the 14-3-3 protein, therefore the patient was diagnosed with sCJD. The patient died 55 days later and autopsy confirmed sCJD.

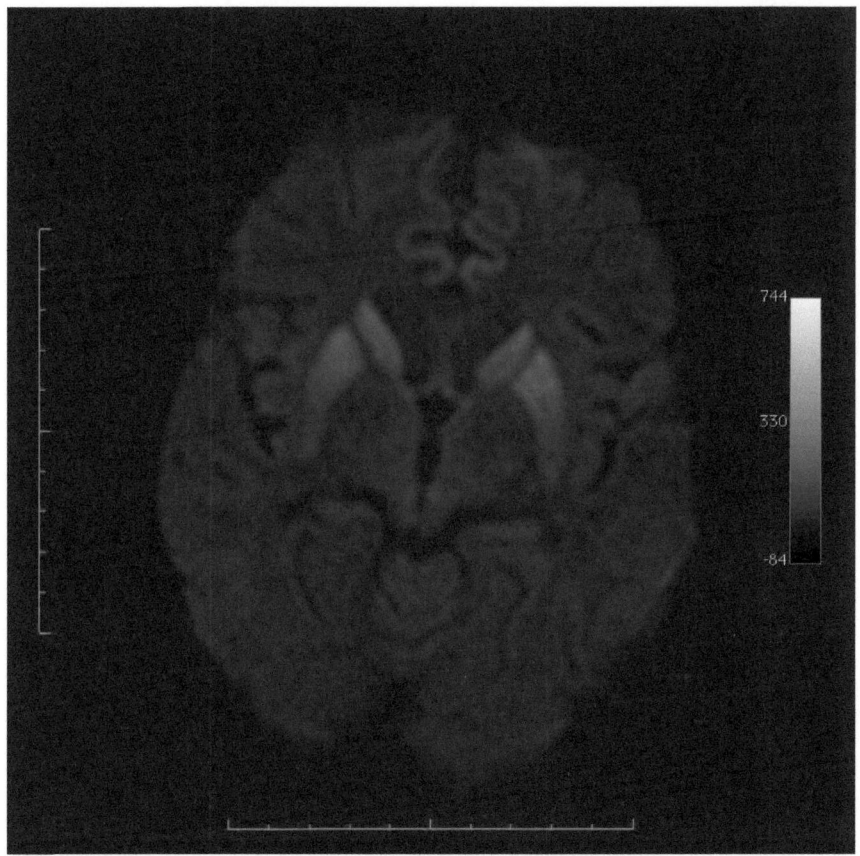

Fig. 9: DWI with hyperintense changes in the anterior putamen and caudate

nucleus.

Case 6

We report a 77-year-old female patient who attended hospital because of

depression and speaking problems.

Clinical examination also revealed ataxia and cognitive impairment.

MRI showed cortical restricted diffusion on both sides concerning the frontal, temporal and parietal lobe. Rolandic cortex was spared out. These lesions detected in DWI (Fig. 10) could not be seen on FLAIR or T2w sequences. CSF analysis was positive for 14-3-3. EEG revealed PSWC. This patient fulfilled the diagnostic criteria for probable sCJD. As the patient moved to another state, there was no follow-up analysis.

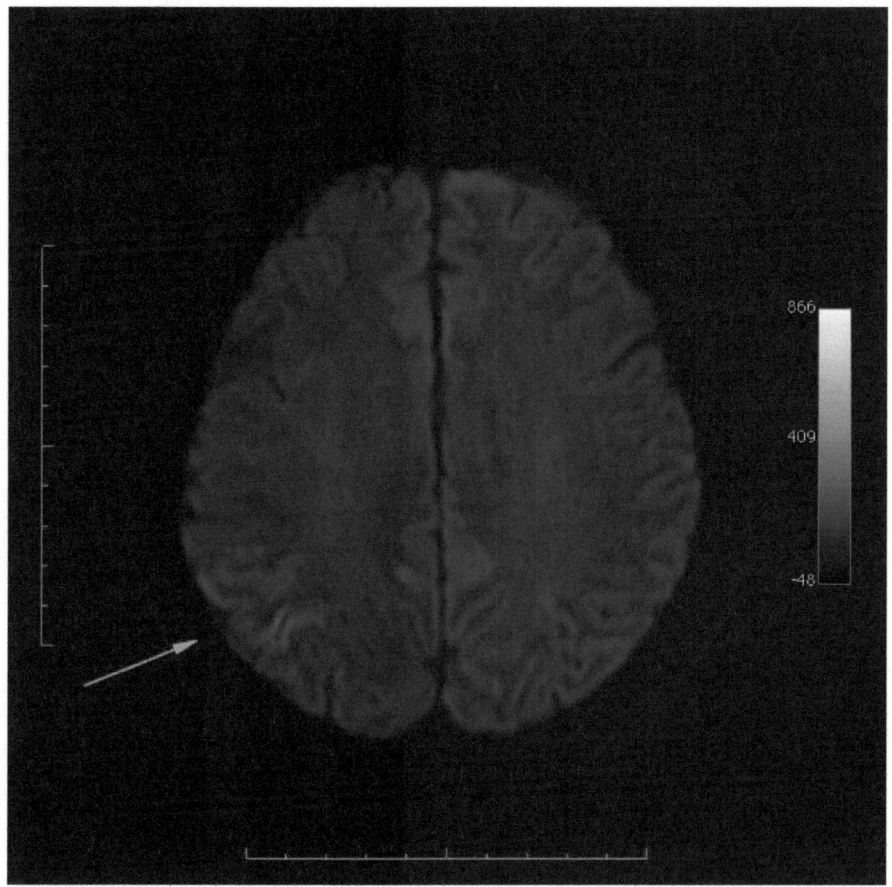

Fig. 10: Hyperintense signal alterations in the parietal lobe on the right side
(arrow).

Results:

Our case series shows an inhomogeneous clinical appearance of disease. Two

patients were initially transferred to hospital because of tremor and one because of vertigo. Four patients came with RPD or altered mental status. The patient in case 4 claimed to have unusual craving for sweet food. All patients had a very fast progressive deterioration in common. In four patients autopsy was available. These patients died 37 to 60 days after the initial diagnosis. All patient samples that were submitted for necropsy were diagnosed as definitive sCJD. The two patients without available autopsy reports were diagnosed as probable sCJD according to the updated diagnostic criteria (7). One patient (case 4) did not formally fulfil the criteria for probable sCJD, however sCJD was diagnosed by autopsy.

All patients showed restricted diffusion in gray matter. Two patients had these lesions only in cortical regions. The other patients showed restricted diffusion in the basal ganglia/thalami. Three patients revealed these changes in the basal ganglia/thalami and cortical region. FLAIR and T2w sequences revealed these lesions just in three cases (cases 2, 4, 5). All lesions with one exception were symmetric. The patient in case 1 just revealed these changes on the left side and even EEG revealed PSWC on the left hemisphere.

14-3-3 protein was positive in all patients except for case 4 and EEG showed typical sharp wave complexes in four cases (Table 1).

The follow up MRI examination in case 4, performed 17 days later remained unchanged.

Case	Sex	Age	EEG [1]	14-3-3	Diagnostic criteria fulfilled	Autopsy after initial diagnosis (days)
1	F	70	PSWC [2]	+	+	37
2	F	52	unspecific	+	+	-
3	M	62	PSWC	+	+	60
4	F	61	normal	-	-	50
5	M	75	unspecific	+	+	55
6	F	77	PSWC	+	+	-

Table 1: Patients´ characteristics.

Discussion

The early, precise diagnosis of CJD is instrumental in order to distinguish this disease from treatable pathologies. The definitive diagnosis requires post mortem neuropathologic examination of brain tissue. To date, the clinical diagnosis has been achieved by using non-invasive tests such as EEG and CSF protein 14-3-3 have been used to aid clinical diagnoses.

The neuroimaging hallmark of sCJD is an increase of the grey matter signal on

[1] Electroencephalogram
[2] Periodic sharp wave complexes

T2-weighted, FLAIR, proton density (PD) and DWI. In most cases MRI shows

bilateral symmetric markedly hyperintense caudate nuclei and putamina,

whereas less common in the thalami and the cortex (7). These lesions might be

symmetric or asymmetric. DWI and FLAIR sequences reveal sensitivity,

specificity and accuracy for high signal changes in the diagnosis of CJD about

>91% (2).

However in early stage of disease FLAIR may remain normal and pathologic

changes can only be detected on DWI (2).

Compared to the study by Zerr et al DWI is more specific compared with 14-3-3

protein (84%) in CSF analysis, while maintaining almost the same sensitivity

(5). According to a study of Mendez et al (8), DWI seems to be more reliable in

the diagnosis among 19 reviewed patients and consistent with this, we also find

one patient with negative 14-3-3 protein but definite sCJD and typical changes

in MRI.

MRI with DWI is more sensitive and specific than EEG (EEG: sensitivity: 64%,

specificity: 91%) according to a study by Steinhoff et al. (9).

The advantages of DWI are its high sensitivity in the detection of cortical

lesions compared with other methods, the time efficiency and the elimination of

motion artefacts in the diagnostic images. It offers high inter observer agreement

and lesions can be detected in early stage of disease compared to FLAIR or T2w

images (2, 7). Another important point is that DWI is well established, available in conventional MRI and therefore standardized. 14-3-3 protein also reveals high sensitivity and specificity, however, the results are not immediately available and it can only be diagnosed in specialized centres.

The pathophysiological correlations of DWI signal hyperintensities with neuronal loss, spongiform changes, and gliosis in deep gray matter structures and cortical regions in sCJD are not well defined and may reflect a spectrum of pathological changes associated with this disease. These include neuronal loss, spongiform changes, and gliosis in deep gray matter structures and cortical regions. Restricted diffusion has been suggested to root in the cytoplasmic vacuolization, which underlies the spongiform changes of CJD (8). It is reported that both, the DWI signal hyperintensities and ADC correlated strongly with neuronal loss and spongiform changes, whereas gliosis was positively correlated only with the ADC. This may explain a related observation that areas of DWI signal hyperintensity develop over the course of sCJD and may disappear with time (10). Data suggests a profile of MRI signal abnormalities in bilateral gyriform cortical and deep gray matter that is characteristic of sCJD and is best appreciated in DWI (8).

According to a study by Vitali et al (11), DWI is also reliable to determine sCJD from other RPD. Diffusion restrictions with negative values in ADC have only been detected in sCJD and have never been present in other RPD (11), highlighting the specificity and significance of this finding. The high sensitivity of DWI in the diagnosis compared to FLAIR, T2w and PDw sequences has already been described elsewhere (7, 12, 13). However, these studies did not address the value of ADC map in initial diagnostic to confirm restricted diffusion. The patient in case 4 of our study had changes in the ADC map even before the onset of symptoms, highlighting the importance of this measure. All of our cases revealed restricted diffusion cortical or/and in the basal ganglia (putamen and cudate nucleus) with or without affection of the thalami. Mendez et al found that in sCJD striatal hyperintensity often reveal a gradual anterior-posterior gradient, involving mainly the caudate nucleus with relative sparing of the posterior putamen (8). These signs seem to be almost unique. However there are noteworthy radiological differential diagnoses. Restricted diffusion in the basal ganglia may also occur in extrapontine myelinolysis (14). However, this entity can be disclosed by blood sample. Other differential diagnosis concerning signal alterations in the basal ganglia are Wilson´s disease, and in the posteriomesial thalamus in Wernicke encephalopathy or Bartonella infection (15, 16, 17). These entities can be ruled out by clinical examination or CSF analysis.

Cortical diffusion restriction can also be detected in the acute phase of viral encephalitis, acute stroke and focal epileptic status (18, 19). Acute viral encephalitis, focal epileptic status, and stroke usually present cortical swelling, subcortical abnormalities, and often contrast enhancement, which do not occur in sCJD (18, 19). Especially cerebral hypoxemia and stroke, which can demonstrate restricted diffusion can be ruled out by a follow-up examination ten days later. While the vasogenic edema at this stage does not show restricted diffusion, in sCJD the low signal in ADC map remains. We also made this observation in the follow-up examination of the patient in case 4 of our study. The hyperintense lesions in the striatum as well as the low signals on ADC map were still detectable and unchanged. In sCJD all regions of the neocortex might be involved with a significant sparing of the primary sensomotoric and visual cortex (20). Also in our cases these regions remain unaffected, especially in patients with major cortical changes (cases 3 and 6).

In regards to clinical signs, cerebellar ataxia and dementia were sensitive and specific for sCJD (21). According to our cases the clinical appearance varies greatly. One patient initially revealed tremor without other neurological pathologies, others demonstrate ataxia and cognitive impairment with changed mental status from the beginning. In one case there was an unusual craving for sweet food. This behaviour may occur in patients with frontotemporal dementia, which is also a progressive neurodegenerative disorder (22). However even in this case, the MRI findings have been typical for sCJD, which was also confirmed by pathologic report.

Conclusion:

We have shown here hat the clinical appearance of sCJD is often heterogeneous and unspecific in the early stage of disease.

We propose that DWI with ADC is a helpful tool in the early diagnosis when clinical features are not reliable. Compared to other diagnostic modalities (e.g. EEG, 14-3-3 protein) DWI is in superior in regard to sensitivity and specificity and it is also possible to exclude other neurodegenerative diseases.

References

1. Prusiner SB Prions. Proc Natl Acad Sci USA 1998; 95:13363–13383

2. Tschampa HJ, Zerr I, Urbach H. Radiological assessment of Creutzfeldt Jakob disease. Eur Radiol 2007; 17:1200-1211

3. World Health Organization. Human transmissible spongiform encephalopathies. Weekly Epidemiological Record 1998; 73:361–365

4. Steinhoff BJ, Racker S, Herrendorf G, et al. Accuracy and reliability of periodic sharp wave complexes in Creutzfeldt-Jakob disease. Arch Neurol 1996; 53:162–166

5. Zerr I, Pocchiari M, Collins S et al. Analysis of EEG and CSF 14-3-3 proteins as aids to the diagnosis of Creutzfeldt-Jakob disease. Neurology 2000;55:811–815

6. Shiga Y, Miyazawa K, Sato S et al. Diffusion-weighted MRI abnormalities as an early diagnostic marker for Creutzfeldt jakob disease. Neurology 2004; 63: 443-449

7. Zerr I., Kallenberg K, Seummers MD et al. Updated clinical diagnostic criteria in sporadic Creutzfeldt Jakob disease. Brain 2009; 132:2659 – 2668.

8. Mendez OE, Shang J, Jungreis CA, Kaufer DI. Diffusion-weighted MRI in Creutzfeldt –Jakob disease: a better diagnostic marker than CSF protein 14-3-3. J Neuroimaging 2003; 13:147-51.

9. Steinhoff BJ, Zerr I, Glatting M, Schulz-Schaeffer W, Poser S, Kretzschmar HA. Diagnostic value of periodic complexes in Creutzfeldt-Jakob disease. Ann Neurol. 2004; 56:702-8

10. Demaerel P, Heiner L, Robberecht W, Sciot R, Wilm G. Diffusion-weighted MRI in sporadic Creutzfeldt-Jakob disease. Neurology 1999; 52:205-208.

11. Vitali P, Maccagnano E, Caverzasi E, Henry RG, Haman A, Torres-Chae C, Johnson DY, Miller BL, Geschwind MD. Diffusion-weighted MRI hyperintensity patterns differentiate CJD from other rapid dementias Neurology 2011; 76:1711-9.

31

12. Meissner B, Kallenberg K, Sanchez-Juan P, et al. MRI lesion profiles in sporadic Creutzfeldt-Jakob disease. Neurology 2009;72:1994–2001.

13. Murata T, Shiga Y, Higano S, Takahashi S, Mugikura S. Conspicuity and evolution of lesions in Creutzfeldt-Jakob disease at diffusion-weighted imaging. AJNR Am J Neuroradiol 2002; 23:1164–1172

14. Martin RJ. Central pontine and extrapontine myelinolysis: the osmotic demyelination syndromes. J Neurol Neurosurg Psychiatry 2004; 75:22–28

15. Sener RN. Diffusion MRI findings in Wilson's disease. Comput Med Imaging Graph 2003; 27:17–21.

16. Chu K, Kang DW, Kim HJ, Lee YS, Park SH. Diffusion-weighted imaging abnormalities in Wernicke encephalopathy: reversible cytotoxic edema? Arch Neurol 2002; 59:123–127.

17. Singhal AB, Newstein MC, Budzik R, et al. Diffusion-weighted magnetic resonance imaging abnormalities in Bartonella encephalopathy. J Neuroimaging 2003; 13:79–82.

18. Herweh C, Jayachandra MR, Hartmann M, et al. Quantitative diffusion tensor imaging in herpes simplex virus encephalitis. J Neurovirol 2007; 13:426-432.

19. Szabo K, Poepel A, Pohlmann-Eden B, et al. Diffusion-weighted and perfusion MRI demonstrates parenchymal changes in complex partial status epilepticus. Brain 2005; 128:1369–1376.

20. Lin YR, Young GS, Chen NK, Dillon WP, Wong S. Creutzfeldt-jakob

disease involvement of rolandic cortex: a quantitative apparent diffusion coefficient evaluation. AJNR Am J Neuroradiol. 2006; 27:1755-9

21. Wang LH, Bucelli RC, Patrick E, Rajderkar D, Alvarez IE, Lim MM, Debruin G, Sharma V, Dahiya S, Schmidt RE, Benzinger TS, Ward BA, Ances BM. Role of magnetic resonance imaging, cerebrospinal fluid, and electroencephalogram in diagnosis of sporadic Creutzfeldt-Jakob disease. J Neurol. 2013; 260:498-508

22. Piguet O, Petersén A, Yin Ka Lam B, Gabery S, Murphy K, Hodges JR, Halliday GM. Eating and hypothalamus changes in behavioral-variant frontotemporal dementia. Ann Neurol. 2011; 69:312-319

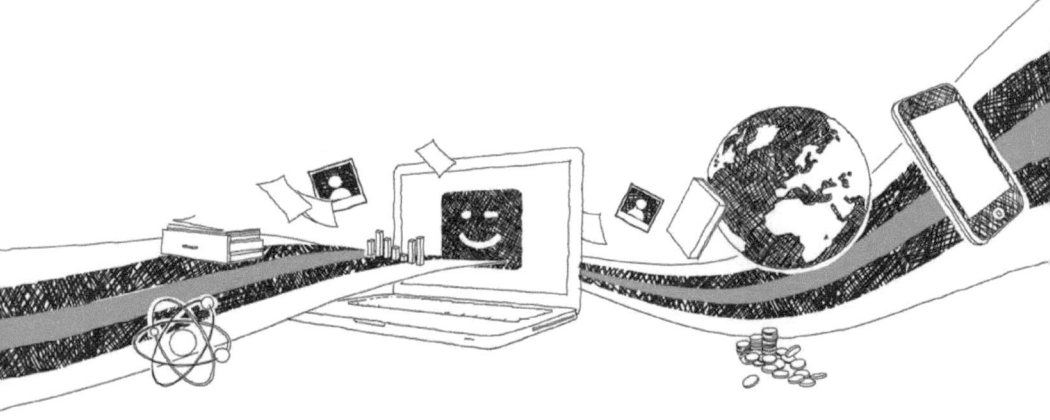
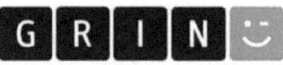